Beating Asthma – The Natural Way To Cure Asthma Fast And Forever.

Stephen S. Reagle

Introduction.

Asthma can there be a cure?
The word "Asthma" seems to have become more common place nowadays. Every year the number of people suffering from it seems to be ever increasing. The World Health Organization (W.H.O) has put the figure at around 150 million people suffering from asthma worldwide, and it doesn't show any signs of decreasing.

As we now know, asthma is caused by inflammation of the lungs. The lining of the lung becomes inflamed and overly sensitive to any foreign body that comes into contact with it. This can come about from stress, exercise, weather conditions, and having a poor breathing technique.

So what can we do, do we just sit back and accept that there is nothing that can be done about asthma, or is it possible to cure it?

Using the natural law of law of action and reaction (for every action there is an equal and opposite reaction), we would see that asthma is an "reaction" of the body, then surely if we took care of the "action" the asthma would disappear. But the way the medical world looks at the problem is that they focus too much on the effect, and don't take any notice of root cause of the problem.

The Common Sense Approach.
If you had a car and took it for a drive, and suddenly the red warning oil light on your cars dashboard started to flash on and off, what would you do?

- Would you take a screwdriver and take the bulb out, and continue on driving?
- Or would you stop, know you have a problem and sort it out?

Or if you had a loose tile on your roof, and you found rain slowly dripping into your bedroom, what would you do?

- Would you go, get a bucket and continuously go about empting it as it filled up.

- Or would you climb up on the roof and fix the loose tile on your roof.

The answer to both of those problems above (the car and the leaking roof) could be solved with some common sense. So why is it then, that we throw all common sense out the window when it comes to our health?

For example when we go to the doctor with our asthma problem (our leaking roof). We're given medication (a bucket) for us to get back up on our feet, and we go away happy. Then as time passes we continue going back, looking to the doctor (to empty our now full bucket), when we should really think about climbing up on the roof and finding the root cause of our asthma.

Doesn't make sense does it?

Your Health Is In Your Hands.
We really should be taking our health into our own hands. In far eastern countries many hundreds of years ago, a doctor's responsibility was to keep a person healthy and free from sickness, if they failed, they were out of work. Nowadays we use doctors the wrong way, we expect our doctors to patch us up and send us on our way.

But unfortunately when we go out the door we return to our bad habits, habits we know deep down are damaging us. You can see this everywhere nowadays, people abuse alcohol, over eat and smoke and then wonder why they can't get the best from their bodies.

But in a way we're being conditioned to behave this way. Everywhere we look and read, the next wonder pill is on its way, and we get suckered in. We look for the easy way out, the shortcut and the drug companies love us for it.

They tell us "If you take our pill, it'll work great and keep your health problems at bay" (not cured now, just at bay, except they don't tell you this.) Then if the wonder drug also has a nasty side effect (which most do), they can always recommend more of their wonder drugs to combat this.

They now have a customer for life, relying on their wonder drug for the rest of your life. In other words you're a cash cow that's going to make them money, right up until the day you die. We can all blame those "big nasty" drug companies for the way their treat us for profit, but at the end of the day, it's all of us that have put them in this position, by falling for the lie that great health can only come through a pill or a potion.

Remember sick people make drug companies money, not healthy ones.

So Where Have Asthma And Our Other Health Conditions Come From?
There is an old saying that goes "It isn't the doctor that cures the body, but nature. In reality the doctor bandages the body, but its nature that heals it."

So where did asthma come from? I believe that as we've moved away from our natural path and started to follow a less natural one. Take the increase in obesity as an example, we've moved away from a proper diet and exercise, and so our bodies have started to become overweight. With asthma and other breathing problems we've moved away from the basics of good health, and taken up some bad habits.

When I say "The basics", I mean the basics of proper breathing.

Bad Breathing Habits.
We all think that just because we breathe every day, we know how to do it, but alas this isn't so. For various reasons like stress, bad posture and lack of exercise, we've taken up some bad habits.

Habits like….

- Breathing through the mouth rather than using the nose.
- Using our chest muscles to breathe with, instead of using our diaphragm.
- Not using the full volume of the lungs, only breathing with the top part of the lung.
- Breathing too fast!
- And finally breathing too much, putting too much oxygen in the body. (Believe it or not, the levels of carbon dioxide in your body are just as important as the levels of oxygen. -More about this in chapter 2)

A lot of people that suffer from asthma have been found to have a dreadful breathing technique. Unfortunately they don't know that by breathing badly like this, they can actually trigger an asthma attack or even make it worse!

So, if you could improve your breathing technique, would your asthma improve also?

Clinical Research Backs Up Breathing Techniques.
It's been well documented in yoga circles that breathing techniques are a fantastic way of promoting better health and bringing calmness in stressful situations, and now there's evidence from the medical world to back up this fact.

In a study done recently in Australia to see if breathing technique could help asthma sufferers. The researchers sought to find out if breathing techniques could make any difference to asthma sufferer's health, and if they could, would they reduce the amount of times rescue inhalers were needed?

Firstly the group was split up into 2 smaller groups. Both groups were asked to try out some breathing techniques given to them on video (a video was used so that the exercises could be performed at home and in a perfect manner). Then both groups were then asked to do their exercises twice daily, working with the video at least once per day.

Group A was told to practice using a shallow breathing technique through the nose for 3-5 minutes, twice per day. Group B was told to do other breathing techniques which included correcting their posture, breathing techniques and some upper body exercises.

In both study groups the participants were also asked to delay how quickly they reached for their rescue inhaler in an emergency. This was to see if they could keep an asthma attack at bay using their new breathing techniques, rather than relying on their inhaler. While all of this way going on, half way through the 30 week trial, the researchers also began lowering the dosage of inhaled corticosteroid in 2 stages.

When the results came back in, the researchers found that although the breathing techniques didn't change their lung functions or quality of life, they did find that the usage rate of asthma inhalers dropped by a whopping 86% and dosages of corticosteroid dropped 50%.

Still Not Sure?
Even if you're sceptical at this point, that maybe using breathing techniques can't help you with your asthma, consider this. If you learned how to breathe better and you had to use inhalers to control your asthma, wouldn't they work better for you if you could inhale deeply? Then at least you'd know that the medication would be going to every area of your airways and lungs, rather than just to the top part of your lungs (if your bad habit was shallow breathing).

So over the next couple of chapters I'll be covering the mechanics of breathing, where we're going wrong, how to correct it and much more.

But firstly ……

Chapter 1.

Where Have We Gone Wrong?
Where have we gone wrong, why don't we breathe properly anymore?
You may not even know you have a poor breathing technique, because
you've been doing it for so long. Some of us aren't even aware that we
aren't using the full capacity of our lungs and our bodies are suffering in
proportion to this. It's easy to see that if more oxygen reached all the cells
and muscles in our bodies, the better our bodies would perform.

The 3 Causes Of Bad Breathing.
 So why has this happened, why have we gotten so bad at breathing, you
may be wondering?

A lot of this can be blamed for these 3 reasons

Stress – We all seem to be under more stress nowadays, constantly
rushing from here to there, trying to get everything done faster and
squeezing as much as we can into our days. (Take the increase in the
readymade meal section of your supermarket, we don't even have the
time to cook anymore.) Because of all this stress we now find ourselves
under, we can get uptight and limit our breathing to the upper chest
muscles with shallow breathing.

The problem with this type of breathing is that it taps into our ingrained
fight or flight mechanism, because our bodies doesn't know the reason
for the shallow breathing. It mightn't know that this is a result of just
being stuck in traffic, rather than being chased by a wild animal. This
stress then causes a build-up of adrenaline which makes the whole thing
worse, and we go on a downward spiral – stress leads to shallow
breathing, which leads to more stress, which leads to adrenaline build up,
and on and on it goes.

Lack Of exercise – We've become more sedentary and now exercise a lot
less than we used to. We all know about the importance of exercise for
building muscle and keeping in shape, but we've probably never
considered the diaphragm (that helps us to breathe) as an important
muscle that also needs a work out every now and then.

Bad Posture – It's easy to fall into the habit of having a bad posture with most of us spending much of our time in a sitting position, either commuting to work or spending our days sitting in front of a computer. Spending our day in a sitting bad position can limit the intake of air into our lungs, which over a period of time can get to become the norm. Unfortunately this type of breathing leads to shallow breathing (where we only use the top third of the lung) which means we use our diaphragm less, use more energy to breathe and lose out on the other benefits good breathing gives us.

Why Upper Chest Breathing Is A No- No!

Being an upper chest breather is bad for us in that, we have to work harder to take in the same amount of air. This is due to the fact that the upper chest muscles are not as energy efficient as our diaphragm. The upper chest muscles were also only built for short bursts of activity, while the diaphragm was built for endurance and is more energy efficient than the energy hungry upper chest muscles. The longer we continue to breathe like this, the more our nerves get used to this situation and our nervous system starts to divert more attention to these muscles and away from the diaphragm. Then as we all know the more a muscle is worked the stronger it gets, and the less a muscle is worked the weaker it gets, thus overtime our diaphragm gets weaker from less use.

But even if we were able to change back to a proper breathing technique, it can take time to build up the diaphragm to its former condition, and undo the wiring in the nervous system to divert its attention from the chest muscles back to the diaphragm.

Can You Turn Your Breathing Habits Around?

Yes, of course you can. Like all habits both good and bad, they were never formed from the first time we did them, but rather they evolved slowly over time. The more they were repeated the stronger they got until finally we now do them without any conscious thought of them.

Take learning to drive a car or riding a bike as an example. Do you remember how awkward and unnatural you felt doing it? You had to give it your total concentration and focus to everything you did, but over time you began to feel more confident and eventually it seemed totally natural for you.

This may feel the same for you, some breathing exercises may seem strange and unnatural but stick with them and they will become second nature. You should also keep in mind that in fact you won't be learning anything new, but rather getting back to how you used to breathe as a baby.

If you're ever looking for a great breathing coach you'll find none better than a new-born baby or small child at sleep. If you watch them as they sleep, you'll notice that all their breathing is done through the nose. Babies from birth never use their mouths for breathing unless they absolutely have to. You'll find they also persevere to use their nose even with a blockage, before they revert to using their mouths for breathing with. You'll also notice that they always breathe with their diaphragm and not the upper chest muscles. You can see this by the way their stomach travels up and down which leads to using the full capacity of their lungs. This all goes to show that from birth we all knew how to breathe properly but because of stress and other outside influences, we've strayed from this path and have got lazy with our breathing.

Now let's take a look at the mechanics of breathing and probably the first mistake that most asthmatics are making.

Chapter 2.

The Nose Has It.
We all have one and they all provide the same function, but do you use yours? As time has moved on a lot of us have moved away from using our nose to breathe through, in favour of using our mouth. This has so common place nowadays that we don't even notice that we're doing it.

But does mouth breathing really matter, surely the same air is still going to our lungs, so what's the problem? Believe it or not, by mouth breathing you can damage your lungs for reasons that you're now bypassing the natural protection of your nose.

The 3 Functions Of The Nose.
The nose provides a 3 different functions.

Warming Air - Our lungs work better using warm air than cold air, and this is an important function of our nose. If you've ever seen any pictures of ancient Stone Age man you'll have noticed that he had a very wide and flat nose. The reason for this being, that his nose had a bigger surface area that could heat up the cold air before it entered his lungs. Try gulping down a few mouthfuls of cold air on a frosty morning and you'll can see how uncomfortable it feels for your lungs and airways.

Filtering Air - We all know the importance of reducing the amount of dirt and debris entering the airways, especially if you have asthma. Any foreign bodies entering the airway can irritate your lungs and airways and can trigger an attack. The inside of our nose is covered in thousands of both visible and invisible hairs who's function is to catch any small pieces of dirt or anything else that it comes in contact with. To further back up this system, our nose also produces a coating of mucus to catch any debris that the hairs haven't caught.

Regulating The Intake Of Oxygen - Because of the difference in size of the openings of the nose compared to the mouth, it's also very important to breathe through the nose. Mouth breathing can cause an uncontrolled level of oxygen to enter into the body, and upset our body's level of carbon dioxide. While we may think of carbon dioxide as a waste gas that just good for plants and trees, it has an important job in our bodies. It's been found that when the levels of carbon dioxide to drop in our body, the body responds by narrowing the blood vessels and airways. In some cases making it harder to breathe which can bring on an asthma attack.

Then why would you use your mouth to breathe through?

One of the reasons why mouth breathing appeals to us, could be that be the fact that we use 50% less effort to breathe through our mouth, over breathing through our nose. Then there are times of stress and intense exercise, when we may feel that we just aren't getting enough air in and use our mouths to gulp down extra air to help catch our breath.

During an asthmatic attack, sufferers can feel that they aren't getting in enough oxygen, but in clinical trials it's been found that most asthmatics already had 100% oxygen saturation in their blood cells already. So no amount of mouth breathing, would ever be able to bring in any more oxygen. It also makes the situation worse, by forcing out too much carbon dioxide and causing the airways to contract even further.

But What If You Have A Blocked Nose?
If you haven't been using your nose as much as you should, you may find it a little blocked. The reason for this, is that repeated breathing through the nose has a cleaning effect and stops the build-up of any debris.

Salt water is a cheap and very effective way of keeping the nasal passage clean. Try the following preparation and you'll have a very effective and cheap nose cleaning mixture....

1. Firstly dissolve half a teaspoon of salt (rock or sea salt) and half a teaspoon of bicarbonate of soda in half a litre of boiled water.

2. Stir the mixture well and allow it to cool.

3. Fill an old sterilized nasal spray bottle or bulb syringe, and spray the back of the nose trying to cover all areas as you do so. Continue to spray until you feel it hit the back of the throat. Sniff gently as you do this and finally clear your throat and spit out any excess water. Do this twice a day, morning and night for 2-3 days and you'll notice a big difference.

If you can't get your hands on a nasal spray bottle, you can use the same mixture and inhale it from the palm of your hand. Close one nostril and inhale the water up into the other open nostril. It can be a bit messy, and you'll find that you may inhale a lot more water than you need, but you'll find that the water will travel far up into your sinuses helping to clear this area. Stick with this procedure (either open palm or nasal spray) and you'll find it will really pay off with a clearer nose to breathe through.

Another nose cleaning method you can use, (if the thought of inhaling salt water seems off putting) is to try inhaling steam over a bowl of off the boil water. To use this technique just place your head above the rising steam and allow it to open up you nasal passage and cavities. You can also add some "Eucalyptus" essential oil to the boiling water to further increase the clearing effect.

Even More Reasons To Breathe Through Your Nostrils.
*Research has shown that our brain is split up into two different parts; the left side of the brain which controls the right side of the body and the processes of thinking speaking and writing. Then the right side of the brain which controls the left part of the body, and the creative parts of the brain that are used for design, art, intuition and imagination.

But as we go through our day and use either the left side or the right side of our brain, our breathing patterns change to suit and we breathe through either the right hand nostril or left hand nostril.

So what does this mean to you?

If you close off one nostril with your finger and try breathing through the opposite nostril for approximately 15 minutes you can change your state of mind. You can go to either a more creative state or a more logical state.

For example if you had an exam coming up, and want to put yourself in the right state of mind. All you would have to do is close off your right nostril and breathe through the opposite nostril you should be in a better state to deal with it. Do you need to do something creative? Just do the same process but block the opposite nostril, and this should help you to open up your creative mind.

This type of research has been backed up by the teachings of Yogis, who discovered the importance of breathing through different nostrils. Which they found could change the temperature of their bodies. The right nostril breathing would cause an increase in body heat and the left nostril breathing could reduce body temperature.

*(This technique was researched by the University of California in San Diego. They found a big increase in brain activity on the same side as the nostril that was being used.)

Chapter 3.

The Diaphragm.
What do you know about the diaphragm, or do you even consider it when you breathe, probably not? Although the lungs get all the accolades and are thought of as how we breathe, if it wasn't for the diaphragm they would just be 2 empty sacks.

You may know the basics of the diaphragm in that it goes up and down like a giant syringe, but we never give the diaphragm any consideration. After the heart, the diaphragm is the second most important muscle in the body. We mightn't be able to see it, or feel it, and yet it pumps up and down between 15-23,000 times per day!

The diaphragm can be found just under the lungs, and separates the lungs from the gut. The diaphragm works by traveling down into the stomach area, the stomach muscles relax and expand to allow this to happen. This action then gently causes a vacuum, which makes the lungs to expand and fill up with air. Then when the lungs are ready to be emptied, the diaphragm is allowed to travel back up as the stomach muscles tighten and force it back up. As you can see the amount of energy needed is very low, compared to the amount of effort that's needed when breathing with the upper chest muscles. It's been said that the chest muscles use up to 10 times as much energy as the diaphragm.

When we breathe better through the diaphragm rather than the chest muscles, we can free up a lot more energy in the body for use elsewhere. Add to this, that the chest muscles are only supposed to be used for short bursts and never to be used for long periods of time. This overuse can then lead to discomfort and burning pains in the upper body, with the build of lactic acid.

The Other Functions Of The Diaphragm.
We know it mains purpose is for breathing, but the diaphragm also has added gives benefits to the body.

Lymphatic System - To explain the lymphatic system better would be to compare it to a garbage collection system. All cells are surrounded with lymph and as the cell goes through its functions it produces waste products that need to be collected. The lymph collects these waste products from all parts of the body and ship them to lymph nodes (the equivalent of a city dump). This is where it's sorted and all waste products old blood cells, chemicals and other toxins are removed and destroyed, and all remaining proteins and needed parts are returned to the body.

(NOTE - Just as a side note, to show the importance of the lymphatic system. If it stopped being pumped around the body, you'd probably be dead within 24 hours, this would come about from the build-up of toxins in the body.)

The lymphatic system has no pump to circulate it around the body, but relies heavily on the diaphragm to push it around the body. So the better the diaphragm works, the more efficient the lymphatic system can be, and the faster the pace it travels at. In a study conducted in Santa Barbara, California, deep breathing and exercise were shown to speed the lymph by up to 15 times.

Digestion – The food that enters our mouth travels down through a tube like muscle called the "Oesophagus". On the way to the stomach, it travels through an opening in the diaphragm. The diaphragm gives support to the valve at the top of the stomach and helps to keep the food traveling back up the oesophagus and causing "heartburn". As it travels up and down, it gently massages the stomach and oesophagus, and helps with the transport of food.

Blood Flow – We all know that the heart pumps blood around our body but the diaphragm also gives a helping hand. By gently giving a helping push as the blood returns from the lower parts of the body, it also helps to reduce the strain on the heart.

Now that we've covered the benefits of the diaphragm, how to you stand in all of this...

Chapter 4.

Have you a bad posture?

As we walk around every day we probably don't even notice how we slouch. We may sit in a bad position and then walk around, carrying ourselves by our shoulders instead of letting them hang loosely. You may not notice it at the time, but by the end of the day you find that your neck muscles are taut and are giving you have a burning pain there. This is a sign that the muscles that are supposed to be doing the work aren't doing it and the wrong ones have to pick up the slack.

I never noticed this myself, until I hurt my back and had to go to the physiotherapist. He stood behind me and then told me that I have a habit or leaning over to my right side (something I never even noticed). I know that it's probably down to the fact that I use my right hand side when I'm doing any type of heavy lifting especially lifting my kids (I usually carry the smallest one on my hip so I can do other things at the same time.)

We all can develop a bad posture over time, and it can be such a gradual thing that we don't even notice it. So how do you know it you have a bad posture, apart from the aching muscles at the end of the day. An easy way is to use a full length mirror and watch how you stand. (If you can't get your hands on a full length mirror, ask someone you trust for their opinion.)

If you're standing correctly your body should be line. To explain this better, imagine that you are looking directly down on yourself from above. Is your head sitting over shoulders? Or have you a habit of leaning your head forward? Are your shoulders hanging loosely or are they rounded forward? Are your hips directly over your feet or are they pushed out to the back? How do you stand on your feet, do you put more pressure on your heels or your toes?

You may have gone through this exercise and found that you seem to have a pretty good posture, but how is your posture when you're sitting watching TV, or at your computer at work.

Do you sit forward face pressed up towards the screen, huddled up with shoulders rounded, or do you sit badly on the lower part of your back rather than your bottom. Both of these example cause your body to become too rounded, which doesn't allow the diaphragm the room to travel up and down. Sitting like this also causes you to breathe with the upper part of your lungs, and use the upper chest muscles to breathe with.

Here are some videos to help improve your posture...
http://www.youtube.com/watch?v=uuL1-27Zj0c
http://www.youtube.com/watch?v=jNtHQ293bXg
http://www.youtube.com/watch?v=0xCEJVPWjWc

Chapter 5.

Is stress causing your asthma?
We all know how our moods and feelings can affect our bodies. A feeling of happiness brings up our energy levels and we feel on top of the world. But we usually take for granted how our bodies are closely linked to our emotions, in fact it's impossible to separate both. It would be like trying to cut a slice of water, impossible and because of this each has an effect on each other.

For example you know that if you go through a stressful time (such as moving house) you can find that you can suddenly come down with an illness, like a cold or flu very easily afterwards. It might not be because you had the stress of physically moving your furniture (if you got removal men), but the stress your mind was under had an effect on your physical body and caused your immune system to fall low enough that the illness got hold.

Feelings of anger and frustration can also totally change how our body behaves in seconds. We feel the muscles tighten up and our blood pressure rise. You can try prove this to yourself right now. Close your eyes for a few minutes and bring up images from your memory that were either bad or good, now see how your body changes accordingly.

So what happens if your emotions don't have an outlet? What if they just are allowed to grow and grow? What do you think would happen, can you see how this can affect your health? We all know that our bodies are creating new cells every second of every day, and then disposing of the older ones.

But did you know that the way you feel at the moment each cell is made, can have an effect on it? If you're angry or depressed, this gets passed over to the cell as it's made and remains there. This stays that way until it finds an outlet either through some type of disease, or cleared through some form of therapy.

To some this may seem far-fetched, but the same thing happens when we eat. As we eat food that's either good or bad, it's broken down and is passed on to every cell of our bodies. So for example if we eat candy, every cell in our body albeit small, gets a share of what's in that candy.

Our Bodies Are More Than We See.
To most of us our bodies are nothing more than just a bag of blood and bones. When in fact we should really think of it as made up of energy. Any scientists will tell you that if we look at the body under a powerful microscope, we'd see that as we look closer past the bone, blood vessels, cells, etc. eventually we'd find ourselves looking at nothing, but energy.

Looking at our bodies this way will allow you to see that all negative thoughts, emotions (negative energy) are repressed and buried deep inside. But rather than being totally gone, they cause an unbalance in our energy system, and tip it in the wrong direction.

How Emotional Issues Can Cause Weight Gain.
Recently in an interview Carol Look from www.AttractingAbundance.com (an EFT practioner) showed how emotional problems can affect our weight levels. Using "Emotional Freedom Techniques" (a form of therapy using the finger tapping on acupuncture points) she had helped a lady clear up some emotional problems that she was suffering from. As she helped the lady over a number of sessions, the lady noticed that she was starting to lose weight. When it was talked over, the lady in question found that her weight problem was not due to any medical reason, but because of emotional issues that she had stored up. As she released them using EFT, her weight loss also followed.

*If you'd like to know more about Emotional Freedom Techniques, visit here....http://www.youtube.com/watch?v=VFKVVP8KXd4

So Could Your Asthma Be Stress Related?
Obviously your environment can have a lot to do with asthma, but what about other people who share your environment with you, have you ever wondered why haven't got asthma also? Why is it that some people suffer from asthma and some don't?

Is it just due to your environment, or is it due to the effect of having a weaker immune system. Then if so, why is your immune system weaker than others? Maybe you think that your asthma is due to a genetic problem, which may be true, but could it also be because of the way you deal with your feelings, and possibly how you think?

So what does this mean for you?

How Pretending To Make Yourself Happy, Can Make You Happy.
Because our minds are so connected to our body, there is no way that they can't affect each other. For example feelings of anger, resentment and hate have nowhere else to go, and are channelled through our bodies. You probably notice this yourself, as you get more stressed your body state changes, shallow breathing, high blood pressure and maybe even grinding of teeth.

But if we look at this in the opposite direction, we can also see that our bodies can also influence our minds. You'll know this only too well if you've ever suffered with a toothache. The pain in your jaw dictates how you are going to feel that day, and the last thing you probably want is be cheerful and full of smiles.

Here's a little experiment you can try out to prove this

We all think that when we're happy we just can't help but smile, but did you know that the opposite is also true. Even if you are in a bad mood you can change your mood by forcing yourself to smile. At the time it will probably be very hard to do, but if you keep trying to break a smile to over and over again, you will find that your mood will lessen and you'll start to feel better.

These finding were discovered by two physiologists Paul Eckman and Wallace Friesen, who were researching facial expressions. In their study they wanted to see if it was possible to read people's minds by their facial expressions. Eckman and Friesen studied people under different situations and used their findings to map the muscles of the face that were being used in each expression. Apart from their research on others, they noticed that the expressions they also made were having an effect on their bodies as well.

For example Eckman noticed that when he turned his face into one of anger, his body responded also and his heartbeat would go up an extra

10-12 beats. On days when they left for home feeling poorly, it was usually after they had spent the day pulling a lot of negative expressions.

So how do you show your emotions?

Are you a person that finds it easy to cry, or do you bottle them up and force them deep inside?
Do you have a lot of anger in your life, or do you need to get something from your past off your chest? Take some time now and try to uncover those things that seem to raise your stress levels? Sit down and take a piece of paper and make a list of what gets your stress levels up, is it a situation, person, or a place that to be blame for that negative feeling? Or is there something in your past that needs to gotten rid of, possibly a past trauma or experience that needs to be cleared first. You may be surprised that your asthma could just be a symptom of an emotional problem. Could your body be using your asthma as a warning sign to attract your attention, to an emotional problem that needs sorting?

Is Your Asthma Being Caused By A Past Issue?
In some cases it was found that a patient's asthma started from just one incidence in the past. In the book "The Self-Hypnosis Book" by Cherith Powell and Greg Forde, worked with a lady in her thirties that suffered from asthma. As they hypnotized and regressed her through her past, she uncovered the very moment that began her asthma.

Through hypnosis she told of being three years old and running in to greet her mother; who entered the room with her their new baby. At the time she was in great spirits, laughing and telling her mother her news. But rather than listening to her, her mother scolded her because she was going to wake the baby who had just fallen asleep.

She was so shocked and gasped at being scolded. Instantly her mood changed instantly from one of joy to one of dejection. This gasp of astonishment was to continue in her life unconsciously every time she was upset. She found that this gasping habit got stronger and stronger until eventually, it caused her to have fully blown asthma.

Now that we've covered how our emotional state can affect our bodies, let's take a look at the physical side of breathing....

Chapter 6.

Breathing exercises
So, where do we begin?   One of the first and foremost rules to proper breathing is to breathe through the nose. This is rule number one. From reading the chapter on the nose, you'll realize the difference it can make to your lungs, both from the benefit of warming and filtering the air that enters your airways. As you go about your day it's also important that you pay more attention to how to breathe. Watch yourself and from time to time and mentally ask yourself the following questions....

Is there any time during your day that you find stressful, and does this cause you to breathe through the mouth? Do you find yourself tightening up and just breathing through your upper chest when stress starts to build up?

How's your posture? Do you spend a lot of sitting down during the day, and if so how do you sit? Are your upper chest and shoulders tight or do they hang loosely? How do you carry yourself when you walk, are you stooped over limiting the movement of your diaphragm? You'll be surprised at how you go through your day, you may be doing things you never were aware of.

As a side-note don't get angry with yourself if you find that you are making the same breathing mistakes (like mouth breathing) over and over again. Instead congratulate yourself for catching yourself doing it, and for trying to turn it around once you noticed it.

What The Best Breathing Exercise To Start Off With?
Firstly you need to discover if you have a good breathing technique by doing the abdominal breath exercise. This exercise helps to uncover if you're more of a chest breather than an abdominal breather.

The Abdominal Breath
To get the best results from this exercise you should do it lying down. It can be done in either a standing or sitting position but for beginner's,

lying down is best because you can totally relax and concentrate on the abdomen.

1. Lie down flat relax, and make yourself comfortable.

2. Place one hand on your stomach and your other hand resting on your upper chest.

3. Inhale slowly and deeply and allow your stomach and abdomen to expand to allow your diaphragm to go fully down. (You should feel your abdomen under your hand, expanding like a balloon.)

4. Let your abdomen fall down as you exhale slowly.

5. As you are exhaling this breath, consciously try to bring your abdomen in towards your spine. (This forces your diaphragm to travel up more, which helps to expel all your old breath.)

Note: If you find this difficult.

1. If you find that the hand on your chest has travelled up more than the hand on your stomach, you now know that the breath you have just taken is from using your upper chest muscles, rather than your abdomen.

2. If you find it hard to get your upper chest muscles to stop working when you're breathing, place your 2 hands behind your head (as if you were relaxing on the beach) this puts your chest muscles in a relaxed position where they can't work as well.

3. If you're still having problems and aren't sure if you're doing this exercise properly you can use a small weight 1-2 kg (like a bag of sugar, rice or something equivalent.) Place the weight on your stomach somewhere just below your belly button. Then continue the exercise as normal and see and feel the weight traveling up and down as you breathe in and out. After you think you've mastered this, you can then place the weight on your upper chest and you should see very little or no movement.

As you get a better feeling for breathing this way, you can try to do it in a sitting or standing position. To get the best results you should consider doing this exercise for about 20 minutes a day broken up into 2x10 minute sessions. Its best to do this exercise for shorter periods throughout your day rather than one longer block further apart. The added benefits of this exercise is that it gives you time to yourself and breathing this way also helps with lowering stress levels.

The Whooshing Breath.
1. Sit or lie down somewhere comfortable and do abdominal breathing for 1-2 minutes to get yourself relaxed and your body warmed up.

2. Inhale through the nose but as you do so make a whooshing sound at the back of your throat. (Although this exercise is described as the whooshing breath, the noise you actually make is a "hmmmm" sound deep in your throat.)

3. Exhale through the nose and make the same noise in the throat again.

The purpose of this exercise is to create a stronger air flow in the lungs and to get rid of impurities, plus it also helps to make you more aware of your nostrils, throat and your lungs as they expand.

The Alternative Nostril Breath.
1. Again for starters, do a few abdominal breaths for 1-2 minutes as a warm up and to help you get relaxed.

2. Close your right nostril with your right thumb and breathe in through your left nostril for a count of two.

3. Now pinch your left nostril closed with your right finger and hold your breath for a count of eight. (At this point both nostrils are now fully pinched closed.)

4. Open your right nostril and exhale through it for a count of four.

5. Inhale through your right nostril for a count of two.

6. Close your right nostril and hold your breath for a count of eight.

7. Open your left nostril and exhale through it for a count of four.

8. Repeat steps 2-7 for 5 minutes (you can gradually work your way up to 15 minutes doing this exercise.)

This exercise may seem difficult at first, because there seems a lot to remember, but stick with it. Start off doing this exercise for just a few minutes at first and gradually start to build up the time.

The Lung Strengthener.
1. Do 2-3 minutes of abdominal breathing.

2. Follow up the abdominal breath with 5-10 minutes of the alternative nostril breath.

3. Perform 2-3 minutes of the whooshing breath. As you do this exercise close your eyes and visualize your lungs as relaxing and being healthy and clear. (You can also visualize the air you're breathing in as having healing energy and traveling to every corner and part of your lungs, and healing them as it goes.)

4. As you go through this exercise you can also say some affirmations to yourself.

Note: (Affirmations are positive statements you make to yourself. You only concentrate only the positive in your affirmation. (For example "With every breath my lungs are becoming stronger, clearer and healthier." Or you can use whatever affirmation you feel comfortable saying.)

The Cleansing Breath.
1. Inhale a complete breath.

2.   Retain the air a few seconds.

3.   Pucker up the lips as if for a whistle (but do not swell out the cheeks), then

exhale a little air through the opening, with considerable vigour. Then stop for a moment, retaining the air, and then exhale a little more air. Repeat until the air is completely exhaled.

Remember that this exercise is to be done with considerable vigour, while exhaling the air through the opening in the lips. This breathing technique can be found quite refreshing, when you feel tired and generally "used up." Try it out and see what you think!

How to Increase Your Chest Expansion.
This exercise is very good for the purpose of restoring natural conditions and gaining chest expansion. One of the reasons that some people have a bad breathing habit is due to having a bad posture, this breathing exercise can undo some of the tightness and open up the chest to allow a fuller breath.

1.   Stand erect.
2.   Inhale a Complete Breath.

3.   Retain the air.

4.   Extend both arms forward and bring your two hands together on a level with your shoulder height.

5.   Then swing back your hands quickly to the sides until the arms are out straight out to the side (still at shoulder height).

6.   Then bring back to Position 4, and swing to Position 5. Repeat several times.

Exhale vigorously through an opened mouth. Finish by practicing the cleansing breath. Use moderation and do not overdo this exercise.

How to Stimulate Your Lung Cells.

PLEASE NOTE. This exercise is designed to stimulate the air cells in the lungs, but beginners must not overdo it, and in no case should it be indulged in too vigorously. Some may find a slight dizziness resulting from the first few trials, in which case walk around a little and discontinue the exercise for a while.

1. Stand erect, with hands at sides.

2. Breathe in very slowly and gradually.

3. While inhaling, gently tap the chest with the fingertips, constantly changing position.

4. When the lungs are filled, retain the breath and pat the chest with the palms of the hands.

5. Finish off by practicing the Cleansing Breath.

Can Younger Children Also Benefit From Breathing Techniques?
Well the answer is "yes", a program for younger children called "Buddies for better breathing" was set up in Tolland, Connecticut in 1979. The program began as a self –help aid for kids to avert asthma attacks. In it children were shown how to do sit ups to strengthen their stomach muscles, this would help them to force trapped air out of the lungs when they were in the middle of an asthma attack.

The children at the program above were shown how to do perform a complete breath through the nose and then taught to exhale through pursed lips. Learning breathing techniques can be boring to a child, because they might not see the benefit of them and stop doing them. So the program made up some games for the kids to do as a way of having fun, and learning the proper breathing technique at the same time.

The following are some games that they used

1. Getting the children to do blow painting by putting a large blob of paint on a page and blowing it in all directions with a straw to make a picture. All the while the child is told to breathe in through the nose and out through the straw.

2. Another game was using a straw again, but having a game of blowing a table tennis (Ping pong ball) around a course. Or having the kids play a game of blow football again using a small light ball, all the while breathing through the nose and out through the straw.

Chapter 7

Using Visualizing For Even Greater Results.

For those who haven't heard of "visualizing" (imaging), this is a process of using the imagination to help to bring about what we want in our life. Although the topic may sound "new age", or "out there", the funny part is we all use visualization every day and give it no thought. Some of us may think that's it only an activity kid's use in the playground, but we can just be as creative.

We imagine scenarios where the worst things can happen to us, our day going badly, what if that car had have hit me, when haven't they phoned, they're late? All of these negative thoughts and visions of doom and gloom can affect us and our bodies. So why not use this power in the reverse, why not use its power to help heal us, and reduce stress levels in our lives.

But wait a minute, I hear you say, what's all of this got to do with my asthma? Please bear with me while I explain. Firstly I want you to try out an exercise for me. Close your eyes and relax, (but until after you've read the following paragraphs), now picture a bowl of fruit on a table in front of you. This bowl is filled with apples grapes and oranges. The oranges look delicious and you take one in your hand. Now slowly feel the orange. It looks delicious and juicy and you can feel the firmness of the fruit inside. Now start to peel the skin off slowly. As you put your finger through the skin some of the juice breaks free, and runs down your finger. Now that you've peeled every piece of skin off the fruit, the soft inside looks delicious. Now I want you to tear a segment off, place it in your mouth and chew it. You can feel the juice fill your mouth as you chew the orange and tanginess sends your taste buds into overdrive.

Now as you visualised this situation, or maybe even as you read the last paragraph your mouth watered? Now think, that orange didn't exist, in fact it's only in this page and in your mind, but it still made your mouth water, didn't it? An imaginary orange still produced a physical effect. We find that our body can react to an image even if the image is a false one. Picture a bad or stressful image and the body reacts, muscles tighten, blood flow is restricted and our blood pressure goes up accordingly.

But if we relax and imagine good or positive images, our body also reacts, but in a positive way. The blood pressure goes down and we can breathe more deeply and fully. Although breathing techniques will relax and bring positive changes in our bodies, we also know that a mind that's full of stressed out or worrying thoughts will never get the best results we're looking for. Also if the thought of doing breathing exercises every day seems boring and tedious, using visualizing techniques you can help freshen it up. This way every session doesn't feel the same and we can come back to it again and again, without feeling bored.

Another benefit of using visualization during breathing exercises is that, we can use imagery to guide us. Although we can't see the lungs and other internal organs as they go about their daily work, we can use our imagination to picture them in action. This helps to focus and pinpoint our attention and energy on that specific body part.

How Visualization Can Affect Your Body.
To better explain this, let's look at a study that was done on a lady that had very poor movement in her intestines. To improve the situation, she was told to hold the image of her intestines as becoming a moving river, flowing smoothly and cleansing on its way. As she held this thought for a while, she was put under a fluoroscope machine (a machine like an x-ray machine, but one where the image can be watched live on monitor). The results of her visualizing showed the image she held in her mind had worked also on her body. Her intestines were working smoothly and full of life, even though she had no sensation of it at all.

So how do you visualize, and what's the best way to do it?

You may be thinking that visualization involves you being able to close your eyes and then have a crystal clear image in your mind. (Like the equivalent of sitting in front of a cinema screen, and having crystal images up in front of you). But this isn't always true.

Some people are more visually orientated, and can conjure images very easily in their minds, while others are more auditory (sound), and then others are kinaesthetically orientated (touch and feeling). If you find it hard to bring up images in your mind don't worry, there's no wrong way to do visualization. If you find sounds or feelings easier to produce then go with that.

For example, if you were to close your eyes right now and think of being in your favourite holiday resort. How would that event or place come to you? Is it the sound of the waves crashing on the beach (auditory), the feeling of a fresh breeze blowing on your face (kinaesthetic) or is it the boats and yachts bobbing on the water (visual)?

By doing this simple exercise you'll uncover, which way you are oriented. Don't be surprised if you can do all three, but all of us are different. Just see what comes easily to you and don't force yourself in the other areas that you're weaker in. Remember visualization is best done in a relaxed state and forcing it will only work against you, and just make things worse.

How Do You Use Visualization And Breathing Exercises Together?
When doing your breathing exercises, you will find that your body will naturally start to relax. At this point you can start to use your visualization, to help you relax even more. Try to find a memory or place that brings you thoughts and feelings of total relaxation. Now bring up all the feelings, images or sounds from that time.

As you do this you will find that your body will enter an even more relaxed state, with the added benefit that it gives your mind something to do. Now as you go through your session of breathing exercise in a very relaxed state, you can now use your visualization on your lungs. As I wrote earlier we can't physically see our internal organs so visualization gives us a target for our focus.

We all know that the lungs can be compared to a pair of balloons that inflate and deflate as they take in air, but why limit yourself to just this image. You can try out the following idea's...

- Picture your lungs as now being strong, healthy and free from any restrictions.
- If you feel that you're not using your lungs to full capacity, you then could picture them as filling up to a greater capacity than before. With each breath being inhaled traveling to every area of the lungs.

- Picture every breath that you inhale as being filled with a white healing energy, which heals and calms all the inflamed and sensitive areas.

You may come up with other ideas or images you would like to try out, there are no restrictions on you. I don't want you to feel that you have to follow these guidelines to the letter, these are only guidelines and you may come up with ideas or techniques that suit you better. Also remember using visualization you can't do any harm to yourself, so don't be afraid to let your imagination go wild.

Using Affirmations To Improve Your Health.
For anyone who hasn't come across the topic of affirmations before, an affirmation is a positive statement that's repeated over and over to reprogram your subconscious mind. For example a health affirmation would be something like "Every day in every way, I'm getting better and better!"

Affirmations are a great way to reprogram all the negative mind chatter we have running around our heads. Most of this mind chatter, is actually old programming and thoughts we've had from our past that we replay over and over again. Negative comments, bad feelings we have about ourselves, comments parents and teachers have made, and everything usually negative affects how we behave and thing about ourselves. These messages form the basis of how we experience the world, and what we think that we can do.

For example you may have some self-defeating thoughts about yourself like "I'm always going to have asthma" "Everyone in my family had asthma, so that's why I have it too" "I'm no good at sport because I'm an asthmatic" and so on and so on. You might think it, but all this negative self-defeating thoughts and mind chatter, can have a negative effect on your health. You may be thinking at this stage, what does this have to do with me and helping me with my asthma. So how does the way I speak to myself mentally, have any bearing on my physical condition?

I'll give you an example of this at work; a number of years ago I used to be involved with a network marketing company which sold nutritional products. At one of our monthly meetings, one of my friend's (Fergus) was taken up to the front of the room to show an example of how the way you talk to ourselves has an effect on us physically.

In an exercise, Fergus was asked to stretch out one of his arms straight to the side (parallel to the floor). After Fergus had done this, he was told to say to himself over and over out loud, "I am weak"… "I am weak"…. for about one minute.

At the end of the minute (Philip the gentlemen hosting the meeting), placed two of his fingers on the back of Fergus's hand and tried to push Fergus's hand down to his side with a little force. All the while Fergus was told to resist this force. All most instantly, Philip pushed Fergus's hand down to his side with very little effort.

This exercise was repeated again, but this time Fergus was asked to repeat over and over "I am strong"… "I am strong" for about the same amount of time. Philip then using the same hand and the same amount of force, tried to press Fergus's hand down again. BUT this time, Fergus's was able to keep his arm in position and resist the force on it.

You can try this experiment yourself if you like, try saying something negative to yourself like, "I am weak" …." I am tired" over and over again for a minute or two. How do you feel? Now try the same thing but this time say something positive like, "I am strong"… "I am full of energy".

Now how did you feel physically on the first part, the negative round? Where you down, did you feel drained? How about on the second positive round, did you feel stronger and more positive? Now imagine the effects of saying those things over and over to yourself, for years and years at a time, because of bad programming (mind chatter). How do you think of yourself, do you see yourself as an asthmatic? Do you live your life through this label? Does everyone know you as "John" or "Jane the asthmatic?"

Now don't get me wrong I'm not saying this to be mean or belittle you, but just as an example to show you, that the way you think of yourself mentally, also has an effect on you physically.
For example in a past job I used to work in, there was one employee John that loved pulling practical jokes on everyone. We'd all had enough and decided that today was the day we were going to turn the tables on him

for a change. On meeting John that morning, one of the other employees asked John if he was OK, because he didn't look to well physically. The first time John replied that he was fine with nothing wrong with him. But as the day went on, and more and more employee's asked the same thing of John his thinking and state changed. Whereas he felt fine that morning, John suddenly thought that maybe there was something wrong with him, and maybe he should go home. While some might have thought it a cruel joke, it did prove to me how thinking the same negative thought over and over again (with a little belief) can affect your health.

To take this train of thought even further, in Australia many years ago. The practice of pointing a stick at enemies and saying a verbal curse was made illegal. This came about when most people who'd had the stick pointed at them, mysteriously died, due to the thought that a curse had been placed on them.   Scary I know, but it just goes to show the power our minds have over our bodies.

6 Tips On Affirmations.
- Your affirmations should always be in the present tense, that great health is already yours now.
- They should always be positive talk about the results you want, not the negative aspect you're looking for. An example would be "I can breathe freely now", rather than "My asthma is going way". Focus on what you want (better breathing), and not on what you don't want (continuing asthma). Always focus on the positive outcome.
- It should be short if possible, this way it can easily be remembered and said.
- It should suit you. An affirmation that works for me, may not work for you. Affirmations work well when they just you a positive feeling when they're said. If it seems too far-fetched, beyond you, or not possible it's probably not going to work for you.
- Accept things as they are, but that you want change in your life. Remember you can't change the past and you only waste energy trying to do so.
- Even a small amount of time on affirmations, for example, 10-15 minutes, can undo many years of negative worn out thoughts about you and your health.

As before there isn't a wrong way to do affirmations. The only thing is that they serve you. Here are a few examples of affirmations you can try out.

"I am healthy and beautiful"
"I give thanks now for a life of health and happiness"
"I love and accept my body completely"
"I deserve to be healthy and feel good"
"It's natural to feel good"

Chapter 8.

Improve Your Air.
Have you ever wondered why do so many people like going to the beach, or going trekking in a forest? You may think that the only difference could be the wide open space and quietness and you would be right. But there are also other factors going on that you won't see but that are still affecting you.

Why Waterfalls Are Good For You.
Have you ever heard of positive or negative ions? If you're like the majority of the public you probably never have, but did you know that you're affected by them every day. While the name "Negative ions" may cause you to think that there is something bad in them, you'd be wrong. These fantastic electrical charges (often regarded as the "vitamins of the air) are the reason we like going to the beach and walking along the shore line. You may also even notice the effects of breathing in the air after a thunder and lightning storm the air seems fresher and cleaned.

But usually and in this case for the good (negative) ion we have, we also have a baddie, the positive ion. Positive ions have a draining effect on us, and are linked to a feeling of heaviness, tiredness and if in high enough quantities depression.

How do you feel when you're in an enclosed building or airplane? The more polluted the area we live in, whether it's in a built up city or a work place with poor air circulation. The greater the amount of positive ions you come into contact with.

In the 1940's and 1950's research was done by the U.S Air force as to why so many of their pilots were passing out at high altitudes. Various testing were done with no success, until they tested the air in the planes. It was found that the air contained a lot more positive ions than negative ions, due to the enclosed and metallic environment of the plane. They found that after they installed negative ion generators to produce negative ions in the planes that the pilots stayed awake longer and stayed alert.

Nowadays, we've become more aware of bad air quality. If you've ever taken a long haul flight or spent a lot of time in an enclosed space with a lot of other people, you'll have noticed how the quality of the air gets worse over time. According to the Wall Street Journal "Complaints on poor air quality are on the increase", leading to a lot of hotel chains to consider how the air quality in their hotels has an effect on their patrons.

So, How Can I Improve My Air?
After reading the so far in this chapter, you'll have noticed how nature has a great part in our air quality, so either we need to spend more time in the great outdoors, or if this isn't possible we have to try to bring more of nature into our homes, by bringing more plants into our environment. Plants release the important oxygen that we need and absorb the carbon dioxide we breathe out. Plants also are great natural air filters they can absorb poisonous gases that are given off by furniture and paint in our homes like ammonia, benzene and formaldehyde. They also reduce the amount of bacteria and funguses and also humidify the air.

What Do You Know About Indoor Pollution?
When you hear about pollution you nearly always picture some cars exhaust pipe, or a large chimney stack pumping large plumes of black or grey smoke into the sky, but what could we be breathing in pollution from just spending time at home?
But did you know that your furniture and fixings are all giving of dust and gasses as you use them? Take your sitting room for starters... did you know that your sofa is adding to pollution by producing dust from the breakdown of the fibres in it?... your bed's also doing the same, the repeated use weakens the fibres and they break down to a small enough size for us to breath them in. We're also constantly breathing in house dust which can be made up of skin cells, moulds, bacteria, animal dander, viruses and pollen. So what can we do about it?

Firstly make sure you house has good ventilation, because some of our homes are so well insulated nowadays, the air doesn't get replaced enough. We all know how buildings have improved over the years, long gone are the homes that used to suffer from drafts entering through windows and doors, sometimes the places that you could have got some warm was from sitting right beside the fire. But on the positive side, these building had fresh air constantly circulating and the levels of indoor pollution was never high because it was well diluted by the amount of air being allowed in.

Nowadays because of double glazing, insulation and draft excluders, the air in a lot of modern buildings and offices is very stagnant. The air doesn't get a chance to be renewed and indoor pollution levels aren't diluted. The best thing to reduce indoor pollution is to open your windows for a spell every day to allow the levels to drop. Investing some money in putting some potted plants around the house not only will they brighten it up, but they also provide more oxygen in the house and collect the carbon dioxide, toxic gases and elements from the air.

To minimize indoor pollution, it's still very important to breathe through your nose and avoid mouth breathing, not doing some means you're bypassing the natural filters in the nose and allowing foreign debris into your airways. Which may cause problems for your asthma and a health issue further down the line.

Chapter 9

Asthma Medication And Its Side Effects.
Because asthma was thought of as basically an airway narrowing disease by the medical community, drugs were created to open and dilate the airways and allow the sufferer a normal breath again. The most common drugs being used today, are beta2-agonist drugs (bronchodilators - which enlarge the airways) and corticosteroids (which soothe the inflammation in the airway). The amounts of these drugs can vary for different circumstances. The most common way of getting these drugs into the body is through the daily use of nebulisers (puffers).

But, what do you know of them? How do they work, and are there any possible side effects? Because the human body is so complex every drug we take into our bodies has an effect everywhere. It's like your food, as the food is broken down and assimilated a small portion travels to every cell of the body. Take "Cod Liver Oil" as an example, most people have the misconception that this oil is great for lubricating the joints, but rather it reduces pain and inflammation in the joints. Not only does it travel to and work there it also has an effect on a person's mood, their heart by helping reduce heart disease.

While some drugs do the job intended they also travel to different areas of the body and unfortunately cause an unbalance in our bodies. These side effects are usually counterbalanced by having to use another drug, but then that drug effects more areas than the first one alone and the body goes even more out of sync.

Corticosteroids.
As I wrote earlier, this drug does a great job of opening up the airways when they narrow during an asthma attack. The long term use of corticosteroids doesn't seem to make any difference to the progression of your asthma but only controls the symptoms. The side effects of corticosteroids in the long term is that they can affect the bone mass of the person using them, which then could lead to osteoporosis in later life. Also in children it can reduce or delay growth by up to 1 inch a year.

Beta-Antagonists.
The function of beta-antagonists is that they stimulate the adrenalin receptor in the lungs which causes them to relax and the airways to open up again. According to the American Academy of Allergy, Asthma and Immunology, beta-antagonists is that while they can help in the short term, they make asthma attacks more severe when they happen. Because beta-antagonists work solely on the adrenal gland over time it becomes less and less receptive, and the benefits of using these wear off. Also older asthma sufferers have a higher chance of suffering from heart problems. Asthma sufferers who used up to 3 canisters a month doubled their chances of being admitted to hospital with heart failure, other adverse effects noticed were palpitations and headaches.

A List Of The Most Commonly Used Asthma Medications And Their Known Side Effects.

Generic name: Budesonide
Brand names: Pulmicort, Rhinocort
Side effects: Facial edema, rash, herpes simplex, nervousness, nausea, nasal irritation, dry mouth, hoarseness, wheezing, nasal pain, delayed growth in children
Long term use: Glucose intolerance, psychiatric disturbances, cataracts

Generic name: Beclomethasone
Brand names: Beclovent, Vanceril, Becloforte, Beconaise
Side effects: Irritation of the throat, coughing, hoarseness, candidiasis in the region of the oropharynx or the larynx.
Long term use: Depressed pituitary-adrenal functioning, osteoporosis.

Generic name: Flunisolide
Brand names: Bronalide, Aerobid-M, Nasalide, Rhinalar
Side effects: Nasal burning and stinging, aftertaste, hoarseness, sore throat, cough, wheezing, Candida (yeast) infections, change or loss of sense of smell or taste, nausea, headache, diarrhoea, allergic reaction (including rash, hives, itchiness and bronchospasm)
Long term use: Permanent loss of sense of smell and/or taste

Generic name: Fluticasone
Brand names: Flonase or Flovent

Side effects: Dry nose, nose bleeds, candida yeast infections in the mouth, hoarseness, sore throat, serious cortisol suppression, growth suppression in children, eosinophilic pneumonia, eosinophilic vasculitis, Churg-Strauss syndrome, vasculitic rash, worsening pulmonary symptoms, cardiac complications, increased risk of glaucoma

Generic name: Salbutamol or Albutrerol
Brand names: Ventolin, Easyhaler, Diskhaler, Proventil
Side effects: Suspected to be a co-factor in asthma deaths, tremor, inner agitation, heart palpitation, muscle cramps, headaches, and premature contractions during pregnancy.

Generic name: Salmeterol
Brand name: Serevent
Side effects: Liver dysfunction and damage, increased heart rate, blood pressure, heart beat irregularities, chest pain tremor, nervousness, worsening of bronchospasm (life-threatening), allergic reactions: skin rash, hives, swelling, bronchospasm, and anaphylaxis (life-threatening), worsening of diabetes and lowering of potassium, potentially fatal heart complications.

Expert Warns Against 5 FDA-Approved Drugs- In testimony Thursday (November 18, 2004) before the Senate Finance Committee, Food and Drug Administration reviewer David Graham cited Meridia, Crestor, Accutane, Bextra and Serevent. Serevent was shown, with 90 percent certainty in a long-term trial in England, to cause deaths due to asthma. GlaxoSmithKline, told by the FDA to do a large, clinical trial, begged off. "We've got case reports of people dying, clutching their Serevent inhaler," Graham said. "But Serevent is still on the market."

Generic name: Prednisone, Prednisolone
Brand names: Adasone, Cartancyl, Colisone, Cordrol, Cortan, Dacortin, Dellacort, Delta-Dome, Deltasone, DiAdreson, Econosone, Fernisone, Liquid Pred, Meticorten, Orasone, Panasol, Paracort, Parmenison, Prednicen-M, Prednicot, Predniment, Rectodelt, Sterapred
Side effects: Systemic corticosteroid effects such as hypercorticism and adrenal suppression, Cushing's syndrome with moon face, truncal obesity, acne, psychiatric disorders, menstruation disorders, osteoporosis, muscular atrophy, and other myopathies, hypertension, edema, hyperglycaemia, cataracts, glaucoma, aseptic bone necrosis, pancreatitis,

delayed wound healing, sleep disturbances, nycturia, nausea; gastrointestinal bleeding, dermatrophy, cerebral pseudotumor, congestive heart failure, convulsions, impaired wound healing
*to discontinue use: prednisolone, or prednisone must be reduced gradually if the therapy lasts longer than one week.

Generic name: Theophylline
Brand names: Theo-dur, Respbid, Slo-bid, Theo-24, Theolair, Uniphyl, Slo-phyllin
Side effects: Loss of appetite, nausea, vomiting, abdominal pain, trouble concentrating tachycardia, palpitations, extrasystoles, headaches, tremor, nervousness, excitability, sleep disturbances, gastroesophageal reflux
Long term use: Dangerous complications mostly affect the heart (arrhythmias) and the central nervous system (convulsions) and are frequently lethal.

Generic name: Zileutron
Brand name: Leutrol, Zyflo
Side effects: Changes in liver functioning
Long term use: Liver damage (yellowing of skin or eyes, unusual tiredness, abdominal pain)

Generic name: Zafirlukast
Brand name: Accolate
Side effects: Headache, infections, nausea, diarrhoea, numbness, tingling, pain, worsening respiratory symptoms, liver damage (yellowing of skin or eyes, unusual tiredness, abdominal pain); Churg-Strauss syndrome: can be very serious; if dose is reduced watch for the following symptoms: fever, muscle aches, pains and weight loss.
Long term use: Liver damage (yellowing of skin or eyes, unusual tiredness, abdominal pain)
instances of life threatening liver failure have been reported to the FDA by Accolate patients

Generic name: Montelukast
Brand name: Singulair
Side effects: Headache, abdominal pain, rash, dyspepsia, dizziness, diarrhoea, sinusitis, and ear ache, gastroenteritis, cough, nasal congestion

Chapter 10

Are Dairy Products Causing Your Asthma?
*Although I wanted to write this e-book entirely on the benefits of correcting your breathing technique, I felt I would be doing you a big disservice not to talk about here the link between dairy products and asthma.

So let's start.....

We've all heard the debate about milk and dairy products. Should you take it or not, that is the question? If you listen to the government and other agencies you would be lead to believe the milk was the best thing to happen on the planet, but is this true? When you think about it, what if everyone in the world stopped drinking milk, what would happen, overnight all the dairy farms and dairy producers would be unemployed. I don't know what the number of people involved would be, but I can imagine the number would be huge! So even if it was doing us harm wouldn't it be better to say it was great, just to keep those people in jobs?

What do you think? Now some of you are probably putting up your hands and saying, but I've taken milk all my life and it's done nothing to me, so what's wrong with it? So why should I cut down or even eliminate it from my life? Before we go any further on the debate about taking milk can I ask a question?

Who did nature intend to drink cow's milk? If you said babies you'd be right, but baby cows that is!

Humans were never meant to drink cow's milk, we were supposed to get it from where nature intended it to come from, and that's from our mother's breast. Cow's milk is nothing like mothers milk, in that it's full of natural growth hormones for the baby cow to go from a weight of less than 100 pounds to a fully grown weight of over 1000 pounds after 2 years.

I don't know about you but I wouldn't fancy bouncing that two year old on my knee!

The argument also that cow's milk is full of protein also doesn't stand up. How much protein do you think is human breast milk, take a guess now before you read any further?

You're probably think it's going to be pretty high as this is the point where babies are going to need it the most, but you'd be wrong, the percentage of protein in mothers milk is actually only 2.38 at birth, and dwindles down to only 1.2 after 6 months.

Having too much protein in your system is also bad for you it that it leeches the calcium from the bones, and it causes your kidneys and urinary track to become over- worked and actually causes you to feel more tired. If we needed to drink cow's milk for its high protein, then why don't we all drink rat's milk as this has a higher percentage of protein than cow's milk? The protein in cow's milk is mostly made up of a substance called "Casein" which in a molecule size too big for humans to digest. Along with casein it also contains 25 other additional type of protein in a form not suited to us, some of which can trigger allergic reactions like, skin rash, eczema, runny nose, sinusitis and wait for it…..asthma!

It's been found that when cow's milk is removed from the sufferers diet all these symptoms disappear. Reports have also found a high incidence of asthma in dairy workers and people who work in cheese factories.

As I wrote about earlier the known triggers of asthma are bad breathing technique, stress and anxiety. But the reason for your asthma could also come from a food intolerance's which may be unknown to you. What your doctor may not have told you or may not have known, is that food intolerance is usually the biggest offender.

Unfortunately doctors only do about 12 hours of training on nutrition in all the years of training they do. For example your doctor may say to you to eat more of a balanced diet but if you pushed him more on this, you'd find that they know nothing more about it other than giving you a print out of the health triangle with your daily intake of food stuffs should be. Maybe you haven't you been made aware of this? Has your doctor ever spoken to you about getting tested for allergies?

We've all heard of food allergies the very dangerous, "peanut or shellfish" allergies which can kill in minutes, right down to the harmless "wheat" allergies that can cause bloating and tiredness. You may have even had some friends that got tested for food allergies in the past, and found with just a small change to their diet their health suddenly turned around. Conditions that followed them all their lives like weight problems, skin problems etc. suddenly cleared up. It's been said before the "Flesh is dumb", your body can't talk for itself but if can give us some hints to point us in the right direction about what we should and shouldn't eat.

Not only are dairy products a common allergy for asthmatics, you should also take a look at other things like coffee and alcohol, especially wine. Some people are very sensitive to "sulphites" which are found in wines and bottled beers. Other than getting your allergies tested to see how your diet is affecting your body you should start to write a food diary and take notes of the things you eat through the day and see if there is a connection to them. Not all allergies reactions are fast like ones to shell fish or peanuts, some can be slow acting and you may not be affected until hours or a days later.

Asthma And E-Numbers.
Other than dairy products, a common allergy for asthmatics are the e-numbers and preservatives that are found in our foods and even in our medicines. But what effect are they having on your body?

Here's just a small list of e-numbers you can refer to when you're on the lookout for allergens.

E-Number   Name   Category   Side Effects
E102   Tartrazine   Colour - Yellow and Orange   Asthmatics sometimes react badly. Take care if you are sensitive to Aspirin.

E122   Carmoisine / Azorubine Colour - Red   Asthmatics sometimes react badly. Take care if you are sensitive to Aspirin.

E124   Ponceau 4R / Cochineal Red A   Colour - Red   Asthmatics sometimes react badly. Take care if you are sensitive to Aspirin.

E131   Patent Blue V   Colour - Blue   Asthmatics sometimes react badly. Take care if you are sensitive to Aspirin. Be cautious if you suffer from allergies or intolerances.

E132   Indigo Carmine / Idigotine   Colour - Blue   Same as E131

E210   Benzoic Acid   Preservative - Benzoic Acid and its salts
Asthmatics sometimes react badly.

E211   Sodium Benzoate   Preservative - Benzoic Acid and its salts
same as E210

E212   Potassium Benzoate   Preservative - Benzoic Acid and its salts
same as E210

E213   Calcium Benzoate   Preservative - Benzoic Acid and its salts
same as E210

E214   Ethyl 4-hydroxybenzoate   Preservative - Benzoic Acid and its
salts   same as E210

E215   Ethyl 4-hydroxybenzoate, Sodium Salt   Preservative - Benzoic
Acid and its salts   same as E210

E216   Propyl 4-hydroxybenzoate   Preservative - Benzoic Acid and its
salts   same as E210

E217   Propyl 4-hydroxybenzoate, Sodium Salt Preservative - Benzoic
Acid and its salts   same as E210

E218   Methyl 4-hydroxybenzoate   Preservative - Benzoic Acid and its
salts   same as E210

E219   Methyl 4-hydroxybenzoate, Sodium Salt Preservative - Benzoic
Acid and its salts   same as E210

E320   Butylated Hydroxyanisole (BHA) Antioxidants- other
Asthmatics sometimes react badly. Be cautious if you suffer from allergies or intolerances.

E321   Butylated Hydroxytoluene (BHT)   Antioxidants- other
        Same as E320

E155   Brown HT   Colours - Brown and Black   Asthmatics
sometimes react badly. Take care if you are sensitive to Aspirin. Be
cautious if you suffer from allergies or intolerances.

Chapter 11

Anti-Oxidants And Foodstuffs For Asthmatics.
It's been found that people with a diet that's low in anti-oxidants suffer more with asthma than others than with a high level. So what does this mean to you, well it means that you should raise your uptake of fruit and vegetables. Every food stuff has its own anti-oxidants properties. Peppers, berries, citrus fruit and apples are high in vitamin C. Carrots and tomatoes are high in beta- carotene and fish and seeds are high in vitamins A, E and selenium. In fact a survey was done in the U.K on 1,500 people showed that if a person ate at least 2 apples per week, they had a 22-32% less risk of having an asthmatic attack, than people who didn't. Vitamin C has been found to be a great natural anti-histamine and helps to reduce inflammation in an asthmatic attack.

Omega 3 and Asthma.
Studies have shown that people who are fish eaters have a lower rate of asthma. It was found that the higher the ratio of omega 3 to omega 6 the better the result. Children with high rates of the later (omega 6) seemed to suffer from worse asthma attacks and other allergies.

Zinc and Magnesium.
Magnesium is the second largest mineral after calcium in the body. Magnesium plays many important roles in the body like regulating the heart, muscles and immune system. It also plays an important role in the body to cope with various allergic conditions like asthma for example. Magnesium given after an asthmatic attack can reduce recovery time by half and the need for recovery by up to two thirds. Magnesium has also been used in conjunction to other drugs in inhalers and has shown to reduce the amount if drugs needed.

Zinc has also shown itself to be just as important for asthmatics. In that it helps the body to produce the essential fatty acids that are important to reducing inflammation in the body. It's needed to restore healthy skin and the lining of the lungs, in studies in animals it's been shown that a deficiency in zinc caused the airways of the animals to tighten.

Ginger.

Ginger and other spices like turmeric have been long used for the relief of asthma, especially in the West Indies. They work so well in that they help to reduce inflammation by turning off inflammation producing protein in the body.